DEFEATING RHEUMATOID ARTHRITIS WITH EXPERT GUIDANCE

Ultimate Solution Handbook For Patients, Guardians Or Family To Understand, Manage, Treat, Prevent, Reverse Symptoms And Live Well

DR. POTTER WHITLEY

DISCLAIMER

This book's contents are meant to be used solely for informative purposes. The information should not be used as a replacement for expert medical advice, diagnosis, or care.

The information contained in this book is accurate and reliable, having been verified by the author to the best of his ability. Nevertheless, the author disclaims all express and implied representations and warranties regarding the availability, correctness, appropriateness, completeness, and reliability of the material provided here. You bear full responsibility for any reliance you may have on such material.

For informational purposes, this book may make reference to or mention of certain people, things, websites, organizations, or other names. The author has no connection to, endorsement from, or recommendation for these organizations. The author's approval or validation is not implied by the inclusion of these references.

Any direct, indirect, incidental, special, or consequential damages resulting from using or not being able to use the material in this book are not covered by the author's liability policy. For medical advice and counsel particular to their circumstances, readers are advised to check with experienced healthcare specialists.

The content, materials, and information in this book are subject to change at any time without prior notice, at the author's discretion. The text may contain errors or omissions for which the author is not responsible.

By reading this book, you understand and accept the conditions of this disclaimer.

THE REASON BEHIND THIS BOOK

"Defeating Rheumatoid Arthritis With Expert Guidance" is an invaluable resource that provides a thorough and perceptive examination of the complexities surrounding this crippling illness. A strong foundation was established in the first few chapters, which explained what rheumatoid arthritis is, its causes, symptoms, and the diagnosis process. This book equips readers with the knowledge and skills necessary to make well-informed decisions as they navigate their health journey.

The story deftly shifts to the significant domains of everyday life, illuminating the extensive ramifications of rheumatoid arthritis. This book discusses the overall impact on one's quality of life, covering everything from the physical difficulties to the subtle emotional and psychological effects. Readers can better understand the condition's complexity and the value of holistic management thanks to this nuanced perspective.

This book's dedication to expert insights is among its most notable qualities. Readers are given a road map for efficient and cooperative healthcare by exploring the role of medical professionals, the importance of early intervention, and the adoption of a holistic treatment approach. This section highlights that overcoming rheumatoid arthritis is a team effort, not an isolated one, and provides hope.

By demystifying biologics, conventional medications, and disease-modifying antirheumatic drugs, the investigation of treatment options and medications adds yet another level of complexity. To provide readers with the information they need to make wise decisions about their health, pain management techniques are covered alongside possible side effects. Beyond the conventional medical approach, this book promotes lifestyle modifications that take into account nutrition, exercise, stress reduction, and the frequently undervalued significance of getting enough sleep.

This book is unique in that it acknowledges the value of mind-body practices, herbal remedies, and acupuncture while taking an inclusive stance on complementary and alternative therapies. This book invites readers to investigate supplementary paths that fit their values and preferences by offering a wide range of options. The focus on developing a robust support network emphasizes even more how closely emotional and physical health are related.

This book gives readers the necessary skills to control flare-ups and deal with the difficulties brought on by rheumatoid arthritis as the story progresses. People are given the tools to take charge during times of increased discomfort using enlightening talks about identifying triggers, identifying early warning signs, and putting coping mechanisms into practice. By offering helpful advice on knowing one's rights, communicating with healthcare providers effectively, getting second opinions, and actively creating one's treatment plan, the emphasis on self-advocacy enhances this empowerment.

With its examination of rheumatoid arthritis research and innovations, this book adopts a forward-looking perspective. Readers are encouraged to stay informed and involved in the changing landscape of treatment options by emphasizing current trends, possible breakthroughs, and the importance of clinical trials. Resilience and an optimistic outlook are fostered among those who are currently navigating their journey by the inclusion of success stories and inspirational journeys, which add a motivational touch and celebrate the victories of people who have overcome rheumatoid arthritis.

To put it simply, "Defeating Rheumatoid Arthritis With Expert Guidance" is a beacon of information, inspiration, and support that goes beyond the typical bounds of health literature. It is more than just a book; it is a lifeline for people struggling with rheumatoid arthritis, offering guidance, empowerment, and ultimately, triumph over the obstacles this illness presents.

TABLE OF CONTENT

CHAPTER ELEVEN

CHAPTER ONE

INTRODUCTION: AN UNDERSTANDING OF RHEUMATOID ARTHRITIS
How Does Rheumatoid Arthritis Occur?

The chronic autoimmune disease known as rheumatoid arthritis (RA) mainly affects the joints, causing pain, inflammation, and possibly even joint damage. When the immune system unintentionally targets the synovium—the lining of the membranes surrounding the joints—rheumatoid arthritis develops, in contrast to osteoarthritis, which is brought on by wear and tear on the joints. This autoimmune reaction sets off an inflammatory chain reaction that results in joint swelling, pain, and eventual damage.

Although the precise etiology of RA is still unknown, a mix of environmental and genetic factors is commonly thought to be involved. The disease can affect not just the joints but also other organs and systems. It frequently presents symmetrically, affecting joints on both sides of the body. Fatigue, fevers, and a general feeling of being unwell are all possible symptoms of rheumatoid arthritis, a systemic illness.

There are phases of remission and flare-ups during the unpredictable course of RA. If left untreated, it can eventually lead to functional impairments and joint deformities. To reduce the disease's long-term effects, early detection and intervention are essential.

Reasons and Hazards

The etiology of rheumatoid arthritis is intricate and multidimensional. Environmental factors also contribute to its development, even though genetics plays a major role. People who have a family history of RA are more likely to get the illness, which may indicate a genetic predisposition. The fact that not everyone who has a genetic predisposition will get RA emphasizes the importance of environmental triggers.

Hormonal fluctuations, smoking, and specific infections are examples of environmental factors that may hasten the onset of RA. One major risk factor that has been found to increase the chance of developing RA as well as the severity of the disease is smoking. Moreover, women are more prone to RA than men, and the risk typically rises with age.

The chance of getting rheumatoid arthritis may also be increased by other autoimmune diseases like lupus. Comprehending these risk factors is imperative for prompt detection and mitigation strategies.

Indications and Expressions

Rheumatoid arthritis can have a wide range of signs and symptoms, which makes early diagnosis difficult. Symptoms that are frequently experienced include stiffness, swelling, and joint pain, especially in the morning or after periods of inactivity. Usually, the affected joints are symmetrical, so if one hand or knee is affected, the other side's corresponding joint is probably going to be badly affected as well.

People may develop fatigue, muscle weakness, and a general feeling of being unwell as the disease worsens. RA can affect organs other than joints, including the skin, eyes, lungs, and heart. Joint malformations may eventually show symptoms, and nodules may form beneath the skin.

For prompt intervention and efficient disease management, early detection of these symptoms is essential. To treat the variety of symptoms related to RA, a multidisciplinary strategy involving rheumatologists, physical therapists, and other medical specialists is frequently used.

Identification of Rheumatoid Arthritis

Rheumatoid arthritis diagnosis is made after a thorough evaluation that takes into account imaging studies, laboratory testing, and clinical symptoms. An important part of the diagnosis process is played by rheumatologists, who specialize in autoimmune diseases. The presence of long-lasting, symmetrical joint inflammation is one of the main diagnostic criteria.

Anti-cyclic citrullinated peptide (anti-CCP) antibodies and rheumatoid factor (RF) tests are frequently performed on blood samples to confirm the diagnosis. An autoimmune reaction is suggested by elevated levels of these markers. The fact that some RA patients may have normal test results, though, should be noted because it highlights the importance of a comprehensive diagnosis process.

Imaging tests that reveal joint damage and help determine the severity of the disease include magnetic resonance imaging (MRI) and X-rays. A thorough diagnosis can be made and treatment plans can be customized to meet the unique needs of each patient by combining clinical evaluation, lab results, and imaging findings.

In summary, rheumatoid arthritis diagnosis is a complicated process that necessitates a careful analysis of several variables. For effective interventions to be implemented, which can impede the disease's advancement and enhance the quality of life for RA patients, early detection is essential.

CHAPTER TWO

THE EFFECTS OF RHEUMATOID ARTHRITIS ON EVERYDAY LIFE, Effects On The Body:

Rheumatoid arthritis (RA) has a significant effect on people's physical health, with a variety of consequences ranging from minor discomfort to severe pain. Inflammation of the joints is one of the main characteristics of RA, and it can cause permanent harm and deformities over time.

Persistent inflammation can impact not only the synovial joints but also other organs, adding to the intricacy of the physical consequences. A common symptom of fatigue is exhaustion, which makes even the most routine daily tasks difficult. RA pain is not constant; it varies, and people may go through episodes of excruciating pain interspersed with periods of relative relief. The swelling and stiffness of the joints reduce their flexibility and limit their range of motion. When these physical effects compound, they can seriously impair a person's capacity to perform daily tasks, which can have an impact on their general independence and functionality.

Psychological and Emotional Impacts:

Apart from the obvious physical consequences, rheumatoid arthritis has a profound impact on the mental and emotional health of those who have it. An ongoing state of stress, anxiety, and even depression is brought on by chronic pain and the unpredictable nature of symptom flare-ups. The emotional cost affects not just the person but also their relationships and social interactions. Feelings of annoyance, powerlessness, and sadness for the life that was once thought to be normal can arise from managing a chronic illness, which frequently requires lifetime care. A negative self-image and a feeling of loneliness can also be exacerbated by the obvious effects of RA, such as joint deformities. The psychological component of RA is important and should not be disregarded because it affects the general well-being of those who are affected by the illness.

Quality of Life Challenges:

People who have rheumatoid arthritis experience a wide range of difficulties that go well beyond the realm of the physical, which significantly reduces their quality of life. Quality of life is closely related to the ability to engage in meaningful activities, sustain relationships, and have a sense of autonomy. The chronic nature of RA typically involves a reevaluation of life objectives and ambitions, as individuals cope with the constraints imposed by the condition. The frequent need for medical attention, the potential adverse effects of drugs, and the financial burden of continued healthcare contribute to the numerous issues experienced by those with RA. Adjusting to a new normal, which may involve modifications in professional pathways, social activities, and life aspirations, becomes a hard undertaking.

Managing Daily Activities:

Effectively managing daily activities becomes a primary emphasis for persons battling rheumatoid arthritis. Simple tasks that are taken for granted in the absence of this disease, such as getting out of bed, dressing, or preparing a meal, become sophisticated obstacles. The necessity for rigorous planning to preserve energy and limit joint stress becomes a daily ritual. Occupational and physical therapy plays a critical role in equipping individuals with skills to negotiate these problems and delivering adaptive approaches and resources to promote independence. Balancing the desire for a happy life with the limits imposed by RA demands regular changes and a proactive attitude to self-care. The management of everyday activities extends beyond physical considerations, incorporating emotional resilience and the creation of a support network to negotiate the specific obstacles provided by rheumatoid arthritis on a day-to-day basis.

CHAPTER THREE

EXPERT INSIGHTS INTO RHEUMATOID ARTHRITIS
Medical Professionals and Specialists

Rheumatoid arthritis (RA) is a complex autoimmune condition that necessitates a multidisciplinary approach for optimal care. Central to this strategy are medical experts and specialists who play pivotal roles in the diagnosis, treatment, and ongoing care of persons with RA. Rheumatologists, in particular, are specialized physicians with knowledge of autoimmune disorders, and their involvement is important in accurately diagnosing RA and establishing personalized treatment programs. These specialists harness their expertise in immunology and rheumatology to traverse the convoluted landscape of RA symptoms and progression.

In addition to rheumatologists, orthopedic surgeons, and physical therapists are key components of the healthcare team. Orthopedic surgeons may be consulted for joint damage evaluation and surgical procedures when necessary, while physical therapists focus on enhancing mobility and functionality through specific exercises. The teamwork among these specialists ensures a complete approach to managing RA, addressing both the underlying inflammation and the physical repercussions of joint deterioration.

Communication and collaboration between medical experts are vital to providing effective care for RA patients. Regular consultations shared medical information, and coordinated decision-making contribute to a holistic treatment plan that considers the multidimensional nature of RA. The knowledge of these specialists jointly provides a united front against the obstacles posed by rheumatoid arthritis.

Importance of Early Intervention

The importance of early intervention in rheumatoid arthritis cannot be emphasized. Early diagnosis and rapid commencement of treatment dramatically improve the disease's trajectory, potentially modifying its course and improving the long-term prognosis for patients. RA is infamous for its progressive nature, causing permanent joint deterioration over time. Timely intervention with disease-modifying antirheumatic medications (DMARDs), frequently the cornerstone of RA treatment, can effectively control inflammation and ameliorate joint deterioration.

Early detection relies on a mix of clinical evaluation, imaging studies, and laboratory tests. Recognizing and managing RA in its early stages not only alleviates symptoms but also prevents the development of severe joint abnormalities and disability. It highlights the significance of frequent tests, especially for persons with a family history of autoimmune illnesses or those experiencing prolonged joint discomfort and swelling.

Beyond medical therapies, early intervention also entails patient education and empowerment. Encouraging individuals to seek medical assistance promptly, boosting awareness about RA symptoms, and cultivating a proactive attitude toward joint health are essential components of this strategy. By prioritizing early intervention, healthcare practitioners and patients can work jointly to fight the stealthy course of rheumatoid arthritis.

Holistic Approach to Treatment

The care of rheumatoid arthritis extends beyond the prescription of pharmaceuticals; it demands a comprehensive approach that covers the physical, emotional, and behavioral components of the individual. Holistic treatment recognizes the interconnectivity of numerous factors causing RA, including stress, food, and overall well-being. Integrating complementary therapies such as acupuncture, yoga, and mindfulness techniques into the treatment regimen can give additional pathways for symptom relief and increased quality of life.

Moreover, nutrition has a key role in treating RA symptoms. Dietary adjustments, such as adopting an anti-inflammatory diet rich in omega-3 fatty acids and antioxidants, can complement medicinal therapies. The collaboration between rheumatologists and nutritionists is crucial to personalize dietary recommendations to the individual needs and preferences of each patient.

Psychosocial assistance is another vital component of a holistic approach. Chronic illnesses like RA can take a toll on mental health, contributing to anxiety and despair. Psychologists and support groups offer useful services to assist individuals in coping with the emotional issues involved with living with a chronic autoimmune disease.

In short, a holistic approach to RA treatment recognizes the intricate interplay of biological, psychological, and social aspects, seeking not simply to manage symptoms but to increase overall well-being and resilience.

Collaborative Healthcare Team

The intricacy of rheumatoid arthritis necessitates a coordinated healthcare team to manage its many difficulties successfully. This team extends beyond medical experts to include other specialties, allied health providers, and, critically, the patient. Open and honest communication among team members ensures a unified approach, promoting a full awareness of the patient's needs and preferences.

Rheumatologists, orthopedic surgeons, physical therapists, nurses, and primary care physicians constitute the basis of the healthcare team. Each member brings a distinct viewpoint and set of abilities to the table, contributing to the creation and execution of a tailored treatment plan. Regular interdisciplinary meetings and case discussions promote the interchange of information, ensuring that the patient receives well-rounded care.

Patient involvement is crucial in this collaborative effort. Empowering patients with rheumatoid arthritis to actively participate in decision-making regarding their treatment develops a sense of ownership and enhances treatment adherence. Moreover, patient input regarding the effectiveness of therapies and their influence on their everyday life is crucial for improving and changing the treatment approach.

Collaboration extends beyond the local healthcare team to encompass ancillary services such as occupational therapy and social work. Occupational therapists aid clients in adjusting their everyday tasks to accommodate physical limits, while social workers provide support in negotiating the psychosocial issues associated with chronic illness.

In conclusion, the collaborative healthcare team serves as the keystone in the overall management of rheumatoid arthritis. By using the experience of multiple clinicians and actively incorporating the patient, this strategy offers a more holistic, patient-centered, and successful response to the complexity of RA.

CHAPTER FOUR

MEDICATION AND THERAPY OPTIONS
Traditional Pharmaceuticals:

When it comes to treating and controlling rheumatoid arthritis (RA), conventional drugs are essential since they provide symptom alleviation and decelerate the disease's progression. As a first line of treatment for pain and inflammation, nonsteroidal anti-inflammatory medications (NSAIDs) are frequently used. By inhibiting the synthesis of prostaglandins, which are molecules that contribute to inflammation, these drugs, such as ibuprofen and naproxen, can control the pain brought on by RA. They don't alter the course of the illness, though; their main function is to relieve symptoms.

For the treatment of RA symptoms, another type of conventional drug is corticosteroids. You can inject these potent anti-inflammatory medications straight into the afflicted joints or take them orally. Long-term corticosteroid use may result in negative effects, such as increased susceptibility to infections and bone loss, despite being effective in delivering immediate relief.

Furthermore, an essential part of traditional RA treatment is the use of disease-modifying antirheumatic medications (DMARDs). Examples of DMARDs that help reduce the immune system's hyperactivity and decrease the course of RA include methotrexate, hydroxychloroquine, and sulfasalazine. The goal of these medications is to avoid abnormalities and maintain joint function.

DMARDs, or Disease-Modifying Antirheumatic Medications:

With targeted medicines that address the underlying immune system malfunction, biologics, and DMARDs represent a breakthrough in the treatment of rheumatoid arthritis. TNF inhibitors are an example of a biologic that functions by selectively inhibiting inflammatory pathways. This focused strategy helps avoid joint injury while simultaneously effectively relieving symptoms. Another biologic that targets B cells is rituximab, which further modifies the immune response.

By inhibiting the immune system, DMARDs—conventional and biological—seek to modify the course of RA. To maximize efficacy, biologics are frequently used in addition to methotrexate, a key component of RA treatment. By addressing several facets of the immune response and inflammation, combining these drugs enables a more thorough approach.

Although the management of RA has been revolutionized by these medications, it is important to take into account potential dangers and side effects. Biologics with DMARDs carry several possible hazards, including infections, infusion responses, and changes in liver function. Effective navigation and mitigation of these risks require strong coordination between patients and healthcare providers as well as routine monitoring.

Pain Reduction Techniques:

For those suffering from rheumatoid arthritis, effective pain management is essential to improving their quality of life. To address the various components of pain that patients experience, a multifaceted strategy is frequently required in addition to medicine. To improve joint function, reduce stiffness, and increase mobility, for example, physical therapy is essential. Exercise routines that are specifically designed to target the muscles around afflicted joints can strengthen them, reducing discomfort and offering stability.

For individuals with RA, occupational therapy is an essential part of pain management. Its main goal is to modify routines to lessen joint stress and improve general function. To enable people to perform everyday tasks more easily, assistive technology, ergonomic changes, and joint protection strategies are frequently used.

Psychological therapies like cognitive-behavioral therapy, in addition to physical and occupational therapy, can assist people in managing the psychological effects of chronic pain. Pain perception may be reduced overall with the use of stress management strategies and relaxation exercises.

Possible Hazards and Adverse Reactions:

Though rheumatoid arthritis sufferers experience great comfort from the many treatment choices available, it's important to recognize and comprehend the dangers and adverse effects that may arise from these interventions. When taken over an extended period, conventional drugs like corticosteroids and NSAIDs can cause cardiovascular problems, gastrointestinal problems, and loss of bone density. It takes constant observation and plan alterations to strike a balance between reducing these adverse effects and efficiently managing symptoms.

DMARDs and biologics have their dangers despite their tailored strategy. A person's immune system can make them more susceptible to infections, so it's important to regularly assess liver function to catch any irregularities early. Furthermore, with some biologics, infusion responses might happen, therefore careful monitoring throughout administration is required.

Patients and healthcare professionals must work together to carefully weigh the benefits of a treatment plan against any potential hazards. In the context of rheumatoid arthritis, successful risk management is based on individualized treatment plans, routine check-ups, and open communication about any emerging symptoms or concerns. Raising patient knowledge and awareness is essential to enabling them to actively participate in their care and make educated decisions regarding their course of treatment.

CHAPTER FIVE

LIFESTYLE MODIFICATIONS FOR THE MANAGEMENT OF RHEUMATOID ARTHRITIS
Nutrition & Diet:

A balanced, nutrient-rich diet is essential for the management of rheumatoid arthritis (RA). It is impossible to overestimate the influence of food decisions on joint health and inflammation. Including foods that reduce inflammation can have a big impact on people with RA. Foods high in omega-3 fatty acids, like walnuts, flaxseeds, and fatty fish, have been associated with a decrease in inflammation. Furthermore, oxidative stress—a condition frequently linked to RA—can be fought off by antioxidants included in fruits and vegetables. Keeping a healthy weight is also essential because being overweight can make joint pain worse. By identifying and avoiding particular items that cause inflammation, some people may find relief by experimenting with an elimination diet. Working with a nutritionist can offer tailored advice that makes sure dietary decisions match personal tastes and health requirements. Maintaining proper hydration is equally crucial because it promotes general health and joint lubrication.

Activity and Exercise:

Exercise is a vital component of controlling rheumatoid arthritis, despite popular belief to the contrary. Even though stiffness and soreness in the joints could make exercising seem impossible, the right exercises can help with joint function and general health. Cardiovascular health is enhanced by low-impact exercises like walking, cycling, and swimming that are easy on the joints. Exercises for strengthening, which concentrate on the muscles surrounding injured joints, can offer stability and lessen joint tension. Flexibility exercises, including tai chi and yoga, improve range of motion and reduce stiffness. However, exercise regimens must be customized to each person's skills and limitations. To create a safe and efficient plan, seek advice from medical professionals or physical therapists. Frequent exercise releases endorphins, which have a favorable effect on mood and mental health in addition to helping one maintain a healthy weight.

Strategies for Stress Management:

Stress management is essential to the treatment of rheumatoid arthritis (RA) because it is a possible trigger for flare-ups. Progressive muscle relaxation, deep breathing exercises, and mindfulness meditation are some of the techniques that can assist people with RA in managing stress and lessen its negative effects on their symptoms.

Mind-body techniques such as yoga and meditation not only help people relax more and feel better mentally, but they also help people reduce stress. People can effectively control their stress levels by establishing a pattern that includes breaks for self-care and relaxation. People can also get emotional support by reaching out to friends, relatives, or support groups, which can help them deal with the difficulties of having a chronic illness like RA.

The Value of Enough Sleep

The importance of getting enough sleep is crucial when it comes to managing rheumatoid arthritis. As getting enough sleep is crucial for maintaining general health and well-being, fatigue is a common symptom of RA. Since overexertion can worsen symptoms and increase joint discomfort, it's important to strike a balance between exercise and rest. Better sleep quality helps with fatigue management.

Two ways to improve sleep quality are by establishing a regular sleep schedule and making your bedroom comfortable. It is crucial to pay attention to the body's cues and take pauses throughout the day, particularly when there is heightened pain or inflammation. To help them sleep better at night, people with RA might find it helpful to practice relaxation exercises beforehand. Rest is a basic component of managing RA, and it has a role in both physical mental, and emotional recovery as well as resilience in the face of a chronic illness.

CHAPTER SIX

COMPLEMENTARY AND ALTERNATIVE THERAPIES
Acupuncture and Acupressure:

The ancient Chinese medical techniques of acupuncture and acupressure have garnered recognition for their promise in the treatment of rheumatoid arthritis (RA). Thin needles are inserted into predetermined bodily locations during acupuncture treatments to encourage the passage of qi and advance healing. In contrast, acupressure applies pressure to the same places without the use of needles. These methods are intended to increase general well-being, lessen inflammation, and ease pain in the setting of RA.

According to studies, acupuncture may influence the immune system and cause the body's natural analgesics, endorphins, to be released. To mitigate the autoimmune mechanisms that underlie rheumatoid arthritis, this regulation may be essential. As a non-invasive substitute, acupressure provides comparable advantages by focusing on particular areas linked to reduced pain and enhanced joint performance. Some patients report a decrease in joint pain and stiffness after adding these therapies to their therapy plan, however, individual reactions may differ.

The holistic approach of acupuncture and acupressure is one of its main benefits. These therapies aim to bring the body back into balance by treating the underlying energy imbalances as well as the physical symptoms. Furthermore, those looking for alternatives to traditional RA therapies will find them appealing due to their very low risk of side effects. To guarantee the correct method and point selection specific to each person's condition, it's crucial to speak with a skilled practitioner.

Herbal Treatments:

Worldwide traditional medical systems have relied heavily on herbal treatments, and more people are becoming aware of their potential for treating rheumatoid arthritis. Many herbs are well-known for their analgesic and anti-inflammatory qualities, which may help with RA symptoms. For example, curcumin, a substance with strong anti-inflammatory properties, is present in turmeric. Another herb that has been researched for its potential to reduce inflammation and ease joint discomfort is Boswellia.

Herbal medicines can have varying degrees of success, and each person will react differently. Herbal treatments have been shown to significantly reduce RA symptoms in certain patients, but caution must be exercised when using them. Herbal supplements may have negative effects or conflict with pharmaceuticals, so it's crucial to speak with a doctor before using them as part of a treatment plan.

Some herbs have anti-inflammatory qualities, but they may also help the immune system as a whole. For instance, echinacea is thought to strengthen the body's defenses naturally, which may help with the treatment of autoimmune diseases like rheumatoid arthritis.

However, practitioners should be aware of their patient's medical histories and approach the use of herbal treatments with a thorough grasp of the dangers and advantages associated with them.

Mind-Body Techniques: Yoga and Meditation

Yoga and meditation are examples of mind-body techniques that have become important parts of the holistic care of rheumatoid arthritis. These methods highlight the link between physical and mental health, which may be helpful for people coping with the long-term discomfort and psychological effects of RA.

Yoga, which incorporates breathing techniques, stretches, and regulated movements, has been demonstrated to help people with rheumatoid arthritis feel better overall, have more flexible joints, and have less pain. Yoga's mild, low-impact style makes it suitable for individuals with different degrees of fitness, offering a physical activity option that can accommodate RA's restrictions.

The emotional components of having a chronic illness are addressed with meditation, which emphasizes mindfulness and relaxation. It is well-recognized that stress aggravates the symptoms of RA, and meditation is an efficient way to reduce stress. Those who practice mindfulness meditation in particular are encouraged to remain in the present moment, which cultivates a positive mindset and lessens worry associated with the uncertainties of living with RA.

An acknowledgment of the connection between mental and physical health can be seen in the inclusion of mind-body techniques in the rheumatoid arthritis treatment plan. These methods can enhance current therapy and help improve the general well-being of RA patients, even though they might not completely replace traditional medical treatments.

The holistic approach to treating rheumatoid arthritis includes vitamins and supplements as a means of addressing nutritional deficiencies and promoting general joint health. For example, vitamin D is necessary for healthy bones and may also influence immune system function. Vitamin D deficiency is common in people with rheumatoid arthritis, and supplementation may help improve results.

Flaxseed and fish oil are good sources of omega-3 fatty acids, which are known to have anti-inflammatory effects. According to studies, people with rheumatoid arthritis may experience less stiffness and pain in their joints if they take omega-3 supplements. These supplements may also improve the cardiovascular system, addressing potential comorbidities related to RA.

Osteoporosis may be more common in people with rheumatoid arthritis as a result of inflammation and drug use. Calcium and magnesium are essential for preserving bone health. Together with a healthy diet, these mineral supplements can support bone density and lower the risk of fractures.

Because supplementing might have negative effects from excessive intake, it is imperative to approach supplementation under the advice of a healthcare practitioner.

Furthermore, since every person's demands are different, customized advice based on detailed nutritional evaluations is essential to maximizing the potential advantages of vitamins and supplements in the context of managing rheumatoid arthritis.

CHAPTER SEVEN

ESTABLISHING A ROBUST SUPPORT NETWORK
Friends and Family:

Constructing a strong support network is essential when negotiating the difficult terrain of overcoming RA. Family and friends are the backbone of this support system, and their empathy and support are crucial to the general well-being of a person living with RA. RA affects not only the physical body but also the emotional and mental states. During the highs and lows of treating this chronic condition, family and friends provide emotional support and understanding, acting as pillars of strength.

When it comes to RA, friends, and family frequently play a crucial role as caregivers, helping with everyday duties that can be difficult for those who have the illness. Family and friends' emotional support lessens the psychological toll that RA takes, promoting the optimistic outlook that is essential for successful management. To guarantee that everyone in the family is aware of the difficulties brought on by RA and can make a significant contribution to the patient's well-being, open communication is crucial.

In addition, educating friends and family about RA improves their capacity to offer knowledgeable support. This can entail going to doctor's visits together or taking part in support group gatherings to learn more about the illness. Family and friends can play a vital role in fostering an atmosphere that supports not just physical health but also emotional resilience when dealing with Rheumatoid Arthritis together.

Support Teams:

Building a solid support network is essential to beating rheumatoid arthritis. Participating in support groups is one way to do this. Support groups provide a special setting where people with comparable problems can exchange experiences, perceptions, and coping mechanisms. By fostering a sense of community, these programs help those who suffer from chronic illnesses like RA feel less alone.

In a support group, members can talk about treatment alternatives, provide emotional support, and trade helpful tips for handling day-to-day tasks. As a result of their increased awareness of their situation and the variety of self-management techniques at their disposal, participants in this collective sharing experience a greater sense of empowerment.

Furthermore, educational seminars offered by professionals in the area are frequently held by support groups, offering insightful information on the most recent advancements in the treatment and management of RA. By participating in these sessions, people and the people in their support systems gain knowledge that is essential for determining the best course of action.

Professionals in Mental Health:

The emotional toll that RA takes means that mental health specialists need to be part of the support system. The general quality of life can be negatively impacted by chronic illnesses such as RA, which can cause increased stress, anxiety, and depression. Psychologists and counselors are among the mental health experts who are vital in helping with these emotional problems.

Individuals with RA can learn coping strategies, build resilience, and manage the psychological effects of their condition through therapy sessions. In addition, mental health practitioners offer a secure environment for patients to communicate their worries and anxieties, assisting them in overcoming the emotional challenges associated with having a chronic illness.

Comprehensive care requires collaboration between medical and mental health providers. A comprehensive approach to controlling Rheumatoid Arthritis is ensured, and the general well-being of the affected individual is improved, by attending to both the physical and emotional components of the condition.

Relationships with others are impacted by rheumatoid arthritis in addition to the affected individual. It takes open communication, empathy, and a common knowledge of the difficulties the disease presents to navigate these relationships. Friends, family, and partners all have special responsibilities to play in this process.

To manage expectations and promote understanding among people who are close to the person with RA, clear communication is essential. Particularly during times of heightened symptom severity, partners may need to adjust to changes in daily routines and provide extra assistance. Having this flexibility and sensitivity is crucial to preserving a solid and encouraging partnership dynamic.

Teaching those in close connections the facts about Rheumatoid Arthritis dispels myths and promotes a proactive approach to care. Incorporating partners and family members into medical appointments might facilitate a collaborative approach to condition management by improving their comprehension of the treatment plan and providing opportunities for inquiries.

Furthermore, people with RA should put self-compassion first and be honest with their support system about what they require. When boundaries are set and appreciation is shown for the help received, a positive dynamic is created that enhances mental health in general.

To summarise, creating a robust support network to overcome Rheumatoid Arthritis necessitates a multifaceted strategy that involves the steadfast assistance of loved ones and friends, proactive participation in support groups, cooperation with mental health specialists, and managing relationships through transparent communication and empathy. Through the integration of these components, people living with RA can create a holistic network that improves their capacity to deal with the difficulties presented by this long-term illness.

CHAPTER EIGHT

HANDLING EMERGENCIES AND ADAPTIVE TECHNIQUES
Recognizing Triggers

One of the most important aspects of effectively managing rheumatoid arthritis (RA) is determining triggers. Triggers are things or occasions that can make the symptoms worse and cause the illness to flare up. People with RA are better able to prevent or reduce their exposure by being aware of these triggers. Stress, particular diets, inactivity, and environmental conditions are common triggers. For example, stress has a major role in inflammation and exacerbates the symptoms of RA. People who are aware of the stresses in their daily lives might create plans to lessen their effects. In a similar vein, pinpointing particular foods that might cause inflammation permits dietary modifications that have a favorable impact on the management of RA. It is crucial to work with medical experts to develop a customized trigger identification plan. This could entail maintaining an in-depth diary of one's activities, feelings, and food to identify trends and develop a thorough grasp of personal triggers.

Early Alert Symptoms of Flares:

The prevention of rheumatoid arthritis symptoms worsening depends on the early detection of flare-ups. By identifying the warning indicators that precede a flare, people might potentially lessen the severity of the impending exacerbation by acting quickly. Frequent early warning indicators include weariness, stiffness, increased joint pain, and a discernible loss of mobility. In this process, regular self-evaluation and discussion with healthcare specialists are essential. Regular consultations with a rheumatologist can help detect new trends and modify medication regimens as necessary. Furthermore, real-time data can be obtained by using wearable technology, which tracks important health measurements. This allows people to react quickly to early warning indicators. The RA community's education and understanding of these indicators promote a proactive attitude by motivating people to seek prompt assistance and professional advice.

Pain and Discomfort Coping Mechanisms:

Handling the ongoing pain and suffering brought on by rheumatoid arthritis is a complex task that calls for an all-encompassing strategy. The cornerstone of pain management is the prescription drugs provided by medical specialists, but supplementary approaches are just as crucial. Stretching and mild exercise are examples of physical therapy techniques that can increase joint flexibility and lessen discomfort. People who use mindfulness practices, such as meditation and deep breathing exercises, are better able to manage the emotional effects of chronic pain and cultivate an optimistic outlook. There are opportunities to share stories and get emotional assistance through therapy and support groups. Additionally, modifying the living space and implementing assistive technology can improve day-to-day functioning and reduce pain. To customize solutions to individual requirements and preferences, a comprehensive approach to pain management entails collaboration between healthcare practitioners, people with RA, and their support networks.

Modifying Daily Schedule During Explosions:

For people with rheumatoid arthritis, it is necessary to modify everyday activities during flare-ups to manage the difficulties caused by increased symptoms. The capacity to adjust daily activities to the restrictions presented by flares requires a strong foundation in flexibility and adaptability. Pacing activities and resting first aid in energy conservation and reduce joint strain. Optimizing functionality can be achieved by scheduling activities during periods when symptoms are usually less acute. Assistive items, including joint support aids or ergonomic tools, can make jobs easier that might otherwise be difficult during flares. Fostering understanding and support among coworkers, employers, and family members is facilitated by open communication regarding the impact of flares.

Keeping the lines of communication open with medical professionals also makes it possible to promptly modify treatment regimens to meet the unique requirements that emerge during flare-ups. In the end, adjusting daily schedules during flare-ups is a dynamic process that necessitates continuous cooperation between RA patients, their support systems, and medical specialists.

CHAPTER NINE

EMPOWERING SELF-ADVOCACY
Understanding Your Rights:

Knowing your rights as a patient is crucial to overcoming rheumatoid arthritis (RA) under professional treatment. The basis for self-advocacy is realizing that you have the right to be informed, involved, and treated with respect. Acknowledging their rights enables patients with RA to actively participate in medical decision-making, as they frequently have to navigate a complicated healthcare system.

In addition to fostering a sense of ownership over their health information, patients should get familiar with their medical records so they can identify any inconsistencies or gaps in the information. Furthermore, knowing how treatments and procedures are consented to guarantees that patients can make knowledgeable decisions regarding their care.

This information becomes an essential tool for promoting the best possible interventions.

Furthermore, being informed of anti-discrimination legislation and safeguards against abuse based on medical problems are vital parts of knowing your rights. Discrimination can take many different forms, ranging from hiring practices to gaining access to public services. Equipped with this knowledge, people with RA can confront any discriminatory actions they come across with assurance, guaranteeing that they are treated fairly.

People with RA can interact with their healthcare providers more equally and intelligently if they are aware of their rights. This highlights the value of self-advocacy in the setting of rheumatoid arthritis and encourages a collaborative approach to care while also improving health outcomes.

Combating Rheumatoid Arthritis requires effective communication with healthcare providers as a key component of successful self-advocacy. Having an honest and open communication style guarantees that people with RA get the best information possible regarding their illness, available treatments, and possible adverse effects. Additionally, it promotes shared decision-making by fostering a relationship between the patient and the medical staff.

Inquiries, clarifications, and concerns should all be voiced by patients as they actively participate in conversations on their treatment plans. To communicate clearly, one must actively listen to the healthcare provider's knowledge and perspectives in addition to giving information. By exchanging information, it becomes easier to customize the treatment plan to each patient's unique requirements and preferences, leading to a more individualized approach to managing RA.

Using written communication can be beneficial in addition to spoken communication. Healthcare professionals can get a thorough picture by keeping a health journal that records symptoms, medication responses, and any lifestyle factors impacting RA. With the help of this instrument, trends can be found and identified, allowing for more focused interventions and treatment plan modifications.

In addition, people with RA ought to feel comfortable talking about how their everyday lives are affected by the illness, particularly in terms of their emotional and psychological health. Good communication encompasses more than just clinical details; it also takes into account the whole experience of living with rheumatoid arthritis. Patients can actively participate in their care by developing an open and cooperative relationship with healthcare providers, which will optimize RA management.

Seeking Reviewed Works:

Getting second opinions becomes important in the fight against Rheumatoid Arthritis and is a key component of self-advocacy. Because of the intricacy of RA and the wide range of treatment choices available, it is imperative that healthcare practitioners thoroughly explore various points of view. While having faith in the primary care physician is crucial, getting a second opinion can yield insightful information, other perspectives, and support for the suggested course of treatment.

Getting a second opinion is a proactive step to make sure that the suggested course of treatment is in line with the patient's values and preferences, not a way to diminish the knowledge and skill of the first healthcare provider. Since RA is a chronic illness with a wide range of symptoms, different physicians may have different insights to provide. Seeking advice from an additional rheumatologist or an expert in autoimmune disorders can provide a more comprehensive comprehension of the accessible therapeutic choices, possible adverse reactions, and extended consequences.

Furthermore, it is especially important to get a second opinion when the diagnosis or suggested course of treatment is unclear or complex. It offers a chance to confirm the results of the preliminary evaluation and investigate further diagnostic procedures or non-traditional treatments. This procedure strengthens the role of people with RA as active participants in their treatment by enabling them to make knowledgeable decisions about their healthcare.

In conclusion, getting second opinions when dealing with rheumatoid arthritis is not only a right but also a proactive move toward thorough and individualized treatment. It improves the person's comprehension of the illness and the range of interventions that are accessible, which helps them manage RA with greater knowledge and assurance.

Taking Charge of Your Therapy Program:

Taking charge of your treatment strategy is essential to overcoming Rheumatoid Arthritis. Even though medical professionals are essential, people with RA should be actively involved in choosing their course of treatment. Being proactive, knowledgeable, and involved in one's health management entails taking charge.

An essential first step is to comprehend the range of potential therapy alternatives. When it comes to biologics, lifestyle changes, and disease-modifying antirheumatic medications (DMARDs), people with RA should be well informed on the advantages and disadvantages of each treatment option. This information serves as the cornerstone for deliberative dialogue with healthcare professionals and informed decision-making.

Being a proactive communicator about treatment choices, lifestyle circumstances, and any concerns or side effects encountered is another aspect of advocating for individualized care. By working together, the treatment plan is guaranteed to be in line with the patient's objectives, principles, and way of life. It might also entail establishing reasonable goals and actively taking part in the monitoring and modification of the treatment plan in response to treatments.

Taking charge also includes self-care routines that support medical procedures. This entails leading a healthful lifestyle, controlling stress, and engaging in physical activity catered to personal tastes and skills. People with RA can improve their quality of life and the overall efficacy of their treatment plan by taking an active role in their well-being.

In summary, taking charge of the treatment plan means working with medical professionals to ensure a comprehensive and customized strategy for beating Rheumatoid Arthritis, not opposing it. By putting the patient first, it empowers them and encourages them to take an active role in their health improvement.

CHAPTER TEN

RHEUMATOID ARTHRITIS RESEARCH AND INNOVATIONS
Trends in RA Research Right Now:

Recent years have seen tremendous changes in the field of rheumatoid arthritis (RA) research, which is indicative of a greater attempt to understand the complexity of this autoimmune disease. One noteworthy development is the move toward individualized treatment, which acknowledges the variability in RA symptoms among people. The hunt for certain biomarkers and genetic variables that might forecast the course of a disease and its reaction to therapy is drawing more and more attention from scientists. By customizing interventions to each patient's specific traits, precision medicine holds the potential to optimize therapeutic outcomes.

Investigating the function of the gut microbiota in the onset and aggravation of RA is a major current trend in RA research. Growing data points to a complex interaction between the immune system and the microbiome that affects the development and course of autoimmune disorders. Gaining insight into these complex relationships may help develop novel treatments, including microbiome-modulating medications, to better control RA.

Research on radiation arthroscopy has also been greatly impacted by developments in imaging technologies. With the use of high-resolution imaging techniques like magnetic resonance imaging and ultrasound, scientists can now see joint inflammation and destruction in unprecedented detail. In addition to helping with early diagnosis, this improved imaging offers insightful information about disease mechanisms, which supports the creation of focused treatment strategies.

Prospective Innovations and New Therapies:

Rheumatoid arthritis is a dynamic disorder with a burgeoning field of potential breakthroughs and developing medicines that could revolutionize the way this chronic condition is managed. The creation of innovative biologic and tailored synthetic disease-modifying antirheumatic medications (DMARDs) is one field of active research. By interfering at particular stages of the immune response, these drugs seek to reduce inflammation and shield joints from harm. The search for more potent and focused therapy is indicative of a dedication to raising the safety and efficacy standards for RA medications.

Furthermore, new and intriguing directions in RA research are being explored in cellular and gene therapy. Researchers are investigating the possibility of modifying the genetic material or cells of patients to control the immune system and stop the advancement of RA. Although these methods are still in the early phases of research and development, they offer patients with RA the chance for long-term remission and constitute a paradigm shift in treatment techniques.

Non-pharmacological methods are becoming more and more popular in addition to pharmaceutical therapies. The potential for customized lifestyle interventions, such as food plans and exercise routines, to supplement conventional medical treatments is being researched. The comprehensive incorporation of lifestyle factors into the management of RA highlights a more comprehensive comprehension of the disease as a complex ailment impacted by a combination of genetic and environmental factors.

Clinical Trial Involvement and Patient Engagement:

Through the assessment of novel therapies' safety and effectiveness, clinical trials are essential to the advancement of the field of rheumatoid arthritis.

Patients must participate in these studies to guarantee that the results of the research are both realistic and supported by science. Efforts to improve patient involvement in clinical trials encompass enhanced patient education campaigns, optimized recruiting procedures, and the integration of patient-reported outcomes to encompass the entire range of the disease's consequences.

Patients who take part in clinical trials can obtain innovative medicines that are not usually offered through routine care. Additionally, it gives people with RA the ability to directly contribute to the growth of medical knowledge, which promotes a sense of agency and involvement in their healthcare journey. To encourage broader and more varied patient involvement, efforts are being made to simplify the clinical trial process and address potential hurdles, such as logistical challenges and misconceptions regarding trial participation.

Keeping Up with Advancements:

Both medical professionals and people with rheumatoid arthritis need to stay up to date on the most recent developments in the disease. Making educated decisions about treatment options and lifestyle choices is made possible by having access to trustworthy and current information. Reputable medical publications, where research papers and reviews are frequently published, are one place to stay updated. Patients need to know about the changing face of RA care, and healthcare providers are essential in providing this information to patients.

Online resources, patient advocacy groups, and medical organizations all play a major role in the diffusion of knowledge in the digital era. Accessible forums, podcasts, and webinars are great places to talk about new developments in RA treatment and offer helpful advice. A comprehensive understanding of the disease and its changing management options is fostered by collaborative efforts among researchers, healthcare practitioners, and patient communities.

Furthermore, medical professionals must receive continuing education to guarantee that they are knowledgeable about the most recent evidence-based procedures. Professionals can get together at conferences, workshops, and ongoing professional development opportunities to share ideas, talk about new findings, and improve their knowledge of treating rheumatoid arthritis patients.

In summary, the dynamic field of rheumatoid arthritis research is characterized by customized strategies, innovative therapies, engaged patient participation, and information sharing across multiple platforms. Together, these patterns advance our understanding of RA more dynamically and comprehensively, opening doors for better treatment outcomes and an improved standard of living for those living with this difficult autoimmune condition.

CHAPTER ELEVEN

ACHIEVEMENTS AND MOTIVATIONAL TALES
Real-World Accounts of People Beaten by Rheumatoid Arthritis:

When it comes to beating Rheumatoid Arthritis (RA), true tales serve as rays of hope and motivation. These stories show the tenacity and resolve of people who successfully overcame RA's obstacles by facing them head-on. For example, Sarah's path demonstrates the resiliency of the human spirit. She was given an RA diagnosis at an early age, and at first, she struggled with pain, stiffness, and future uncertainty. But Sarah changed her life, thanks to a combination of professional medical advice, steadfast family support, and her willpower. She adjusted to a customized treatment plan that included lifestyle modifications, physical therapy, and medication that progressively reduced her symptoms. Her experience demonstrates the value of early intervention as well as the transformational potential of resilience in the face of long-term illness.

Positivity and Resilience:

The key to beating Rheumatoid Arthritis is resilience, and having an optimistic outlook is a great motivator in this process. Mark's experience serves as a powerful example of this synergy. At first, Mark was overcome by the psychological and physical effects of RA, so he decided to take charge of his story. Rather than giving in to hopelessness, he adopted an outlook that saw each obstacle as a chance for improvement. He was able to face the difficulties of RA with renewed strength by using this lens. Mark included daily routines with mindfulness activities like gratitude exercises and meditation. Through these routines, he was able to control stress, which is known to set off RA flare-ups. They also fostered optimism, which strengthened his fortitude. Mark's experience demonstrates the transformational power of resilience and an optimistic outlook, demonstrating that addressing the psychological aspect of RA is just as important as addressing the physical.

Inspiration for Individuals Traveling:

Tales of victory are a powerful source of inspiration for people who are presently navigating the difficult terrain of rheumatoid arthritis. Emma, a mid-30s diagnosed individual, personifies this drive. Emma set out on a mission of education after being confronted with the terrifying idea that RA would change her life. By being knowledgeable about the illness, available treatments, and lifestyle modifications, she took an active role in her recovery.

This sense of empowerment gave her the drive to push through the difficult times. Emma's narrative inspires those who are following in her footsteps to take charge of their health, to look for knowledge, and to interact with their medical team proactively. Her story demonstrates how, despite the obstacles presented by rheumatoid arthritis, education, and motivation are unbreakable partners, enabling people to live more fully and empowered lives.

Honoring Wins, Great and Small:

Celebrating triumphs, no matter how minor, is essential to keeping up the momentum and creating a sense of accomplishment in the fight against Rheumatoid Arthritis. Michael's narrative serves as an example of this idea. Every accomplishment, from the early difficulty with routine daily chores to reaching big goals like finishing a 5K, was the reason for the celebration. With the help of his medical team, Michael adopted a methodical yet progressive strategy to take back control of his life.

Acknowledging and celebrating every accomplishment, no matter how small, became an essential part of his path. His narrative highlights that little successes, like pain-free mornings or enhanced mobility, may be achieved in the face of RA. Michael's story serves as a reminder that surviving rheumatoid arthritis is a series of little victories that should all be recognized and celebrated.